Ki Balance
Massage

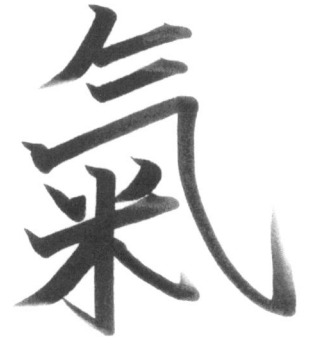

EDWARD ESKO
NAOMI ICHIKAWA ESKO

IMI Press
Lenox, Massachusetts

KI BALANCE MASSAGE

CONTENTS

Ki Balance Massage
Copyright © Edward Esko
Introduction Copyright © Naomi Ichikawa Esko
Photos: Yoshiko Harimaya. Copyright © Naomi Ichikawa Esko
Models: Naomi Ichikawa Esko, Taeka Nagamoto
Title Page Kanji of "Ki": Naomi Ichikawa Esko

ISBN-13: 978-1545269831
ISBN-10: 1545269831

Published by IMI Press
A Division of International Macrobiotic Institute
InternationalMacrobioticInstitute.com
First Edition: Spring 2017

Foreword

Thousands of years ago people understood that the human body was made up of something other than bones, skin, cells, and fluids. The ancients knew that an invisible force permeated all of nature. All living things were seen as part of that universal web. The ancients regarded that invisible force as the energy of life itself.

The force of the universe was given names such as "Ki" (pronounced "kee"), in Japan, "Ch'i" in China, and "prana" in India. These terms are still in use today, as are numerous arts based on their understanding. In acupuncture, for example, thin metal needles are inserted in certain key points to adjust energy and establish balance. The acupuncturist will use needles to channel energy to places that lack it, or from places that have too much.

In Japan, health is referred to as "Gen-Ki," or "original energy," in an acknowledgement that life force is the foundation of health, and also that health is our original state. On the other hand, sickness is known as "Byo-Ki," or "suffering energy." In the healing tradition of Hawaii, good health means that someone has an "abundance of energy." The word for "healing" means to restore energy and achieve a condition of harmony or fullness.

Hippocrates and other Greek physicians were well aware of the life force. They called it "pneuma" and believed that it flowed within and through every person. When the pneuma was strong, a person could resist the natural causes of illness. When it became weak, the person more easily succumbed to the symptoms of disease. Many centuries later, the German physician, Cristoph Wilhelm Hufeland, a contemporary of Goethe, advocated strengthening life energy as the means to health and longevity. In his widely read and influential book, *Makrobiotik*, Hufeland referred to life energy as "Lebenskraft," or "life vitality."

Not only did the ancients understand that the body was animated by life energy, they actually mapped its origins, contours, and direction of flow, as well as its relationship to heaven and earth and the cycles of time and season.

3

Ancient healers perceived the body, including all of its cells, organs, tissues, and fluids, as a complex, interconnected network of energy. It was discovered that energy flows through the body in the way water flows from a river into small streams, in other words, through a pattern of fractal, or yin and yang division.

The simple techniques in this book are designed to help you balance and harmonize Ki. They enable you to help others with basic massage. They represent a fundamental yet effective application of yin and yang, the forces that create and animate life energy. These techniques employ such basic polarities as left and right, front and back, upper and lower, and physical and energetic. The goal is to help each person achieve and maintain a harmonious unity of opposites, as the foundation for the smooth and active circulation of Ki throughout the body. Remember that health and healing are rooted in unity or wholeness. Think of these exercises as basic methods for attuning a person's life energy to the rhythms and energies of heaven, earth, and nature as a whole.

Feel free to apply these simple methods to relieve stress and tension among your friends and family. You can make A La Carte selections from our menu of techniques. Simply apply any one or several of these methods to relieve specific stress or tension. Or you can incorporate them into a full body massage, beginning with the shoulders and temples; proceeding to the back, buttocks, legs and feet, arms and hands, and concluding with the abdomen and face. The sections of the book are arranged in this order for your convenience.

It is our hope that, in addition to a natural plant-based diet and active lifestyle, the basic techniques in *Ki Balance Massage* will become part of everyone's daily health routine.

Edward Esko
IMI Press
Pittsfield and Lenox, Massachusetts

Introduction

In the spring of 2010, I was studying at the Kushi Institute in Massachusetts. During my studies, Shiatsu (finger pressure) massage was part of the curriculum. Actually, for people in Japan, the points used in Shiatsu are quite familiar. But the study of meridians, or energy pathways, was new to me. I discovered that each organ has a related meridian and that meridians are clear reflections of our condition. For example, whenever I ate too much, my stomach meridian became tight and painful. While at the Institute, my Shiatsu teacher did massage on my stomach meridian. It was amazing. Following the massage, my overactive stomach calmed down!

At that time I realized how simple our body actually is. I also realized that we all have natural healing ability and that we can use our hands to heal others and ourselves. In Japanese we say, " Te-Ate." "Te" means, "hand," and "Ate" means, "to touch." So if you have pain, place your hand on the area or ask another person to touch the painful place. You may be surprised to discover that your pain becomes less.

I have found massage to be extremely beneficial in improving both my circulation and overall vitality. At the same time, together with a balanced plant-based diet, regular massage helped me lose excess weight. It also helped me establish a more healthful and appealing body shape. The flow of Ki is very important for our health. I have changed my condition with a plant-based diet and energy work such as that presented in *Ki Balance Massage*. I hope you can use these methods to improve as well.

Naomi Ichikawa Esko
April 2017

Note to the Reader

From Merriam Webster

Ki
Aura, chi (OR ch'i ALSO qi), energy, vibe(s), vibration(s)

Balance
Counterpoise, equilibration, equilibrium, equipoise, poise, stasis

Massage
French, from *masser* "to massage," from Arabic *massa* "to stroke"

From IMI Press

Please note that the exercises presented in this book are for general educational purposes only. They are provided for the basic purpose of adjusting and balancing Ki energy and providing relief from stress and tension in normally healthy adults. Persons performing these techniques need to exercise commonsense, caution, and good judgment. Don't' forget, you are entering another person's space. Be sensitive and respectful at all times.

Persons receiving these techniques need to inform the practitioner of any medical conditions, such as arthritis, osteoporosis, bone weakness or fractures, stiff, painful, or inflamed joints, injuries, or others that preclude the proposed exercise, or if they experience any pain of discomfort during an exercise so that pressure or strokes may be discontinued or adjusted to a suitable level of comfort.

The exercises in this book should not be considered a substitute for medical examination, diagnosis, or treatment. Persons with mental or physical ailments should consult the appropriate health care provider. The authors assume no responsibility for any and all consequences resulting from the performance of the exercises presented in this book.

Releasing Shoulder Tension

The shoulders are frequently a site for tension and tightness. Aside from showing the condition of the body as a whole, the shoulders reflect the condition of the intestines, as the meridians corresponding to these organs run through them. Shoulder tightness is often the result of too much animal food, bread and baked flour products, and overeating in general. To improve this condition, switch to a plant-based diet, reduce baked foods, chew well, and eat less. Try to avoid eating before bed. Exercise more often.

To relax the shoulders, have the receiver sit comfortably on the floor or on a chair. Kneel or stand behind them and place both palms gently on the shoulder muscle. Extend your fingers toward the front and your thumbs opposite on the back. Begin gently kneading the shoulders, working outward from the neck. Continue several minutes or as needed until the shoulders become soft and relaxed. The receiver should experience the melting away of stress and tension.

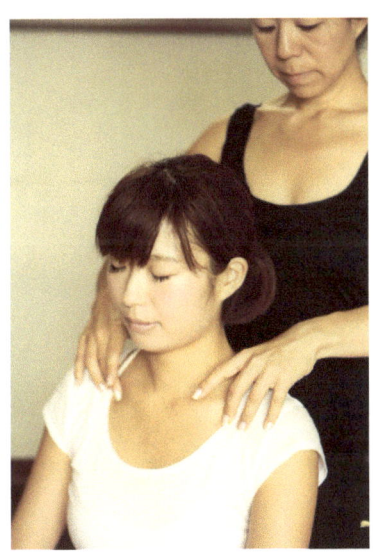

Activating the Shoulders

You can further relax and energize the shoulders by tapping (firmly but gently) with the edge of your palms and fingers. Keep your wrists relaxed and your fingers extended. Begin tapping with an alternating up and down and left-right movement. Start at the neck and work your way out to the shoulders. The kneading motion done previously has the effect of relaxing the muscles and energy meridians. Relaxation and release of tension are yin or expansive. The gentle tapping motion done in this stage has the opposite effect of activating energy in the meridians, intestines, and body as a whole. This more yang effect perfectly balances the yin relaxing effect achieved previously.

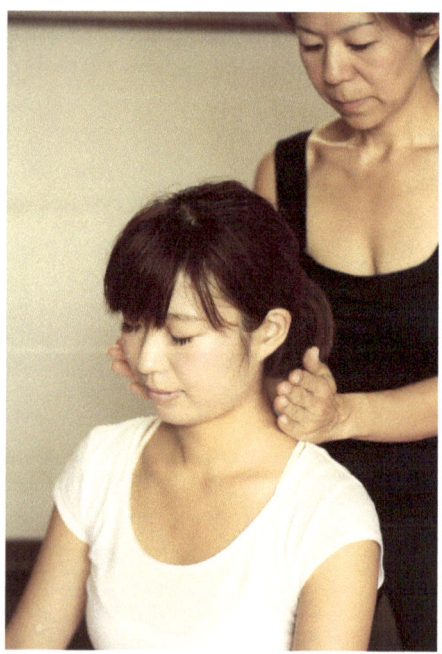

Easing Tightness in the Neck

Pain or tightness in the neck is a common occurrence today. Gentle massage can help ease this condition. Have the receiver sit comfortably on the floor or in a chair. Kneel or stand alongside the receiver at a 45-degree angle. Place your active hand on the neck at the base of the skull, with your fingers to one side and your thumb to the opposite side. Place your opposite hand on the forehead for support. Begin massaging the neck in a gentle back and forth and/or circular motion. Continue until the neck becomes softer and tension is released.

Tightness in the neck is often the result of excess animal food, salt, and baked flour. These excesses have a negative impact on the liver and gallbladder.

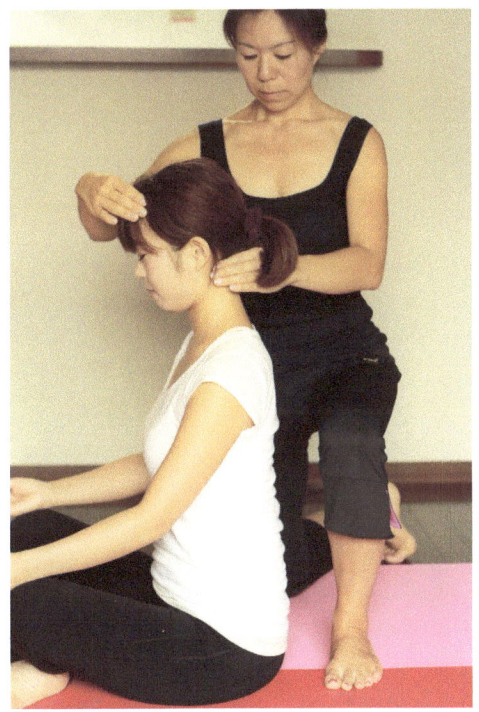

Relieving Stress in the Temples

Many people hold tension on the side of the head. This area is related to the gallbladder. Tension here is often a sign of excess intake of oily and fatty foods. Foods such as barley, barley tea, green vegetables, including dandelion and raw scallion, and daikon radish help dissolve fats and loosen stagnation.

To help relieve tension in the temples, have the person sit comfortably on the floor on chair. Sit or stand behind them. Breathe together and extend your fingers. Place them on the sides of the head and begin to massage using a gentle circular motion. Keep a slow steady rhythm with your hands. Continue for two to three minutes before stopping.

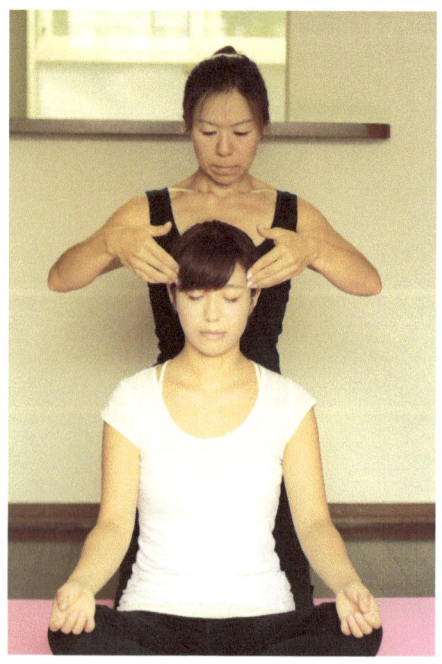

Relaxing the Back

When we massage the back, we are affecting all of the body's organs. We accomplish this by stimulating the bladder meridian that runs along either side of the spine. The meridian runs from the head down to the fifth toe, passing through the back and back of both legs. There are points along the bladder lines, known as "Yu" points, that feed energy to the internal organs.

Have the receiver lie on his or her front with their head turned sideways and arms extended comfortably to the side. Place a pillow or cushion under the receiver's head so that he or she is comfortable. Kneel to the side of the receiver and leave your active hand free for massage. Place your palm on one side of the spine with your thumb extended. Begin to massage with a gentle kneading motion. Start at the top below the shoulder and gradually work your way down to the buttock. Repeat several times and then do the same on the opposite side. When you finish, gently brush down one side and then the other, repeating several times so as to calm, soothe, and ultimately relax the person's energy.

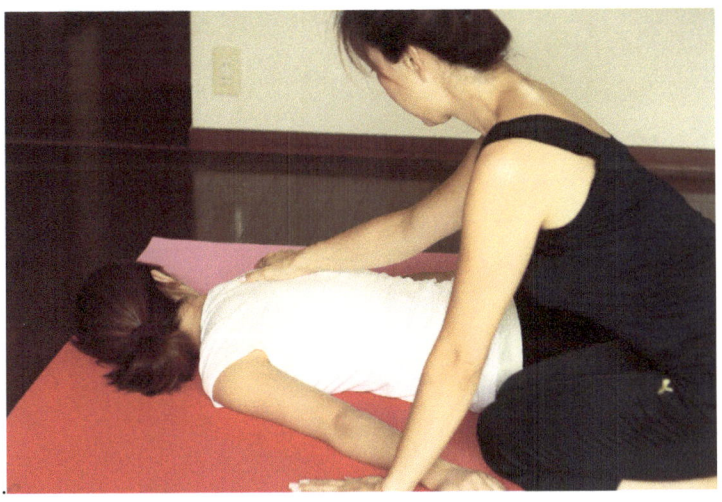

Soothing the Spine

The governing vessel meridian runs along the center of the spine. It energies the entire body, especially the nervous system and spine, and is a conduit for energy reaching the body's energy centers, or chakras, from the outside. When we masage the spine, we are especially energizing and stimuating the heart chakra in the chest, the stomach chakra in the solar plexus, and the small intestine, or hara chakra in the lower abdomen.

From a kneeling postion alongside the receiver, place your active hand on the spine and place your other hand on top. Begin at the upper spine. Coordinate your breathing. As you exhale together, gently press downward. Lean forward slightly as you press. Inhale and release pressure. Repeat down the entire length of the spine to the tailbone. Repeat several times.

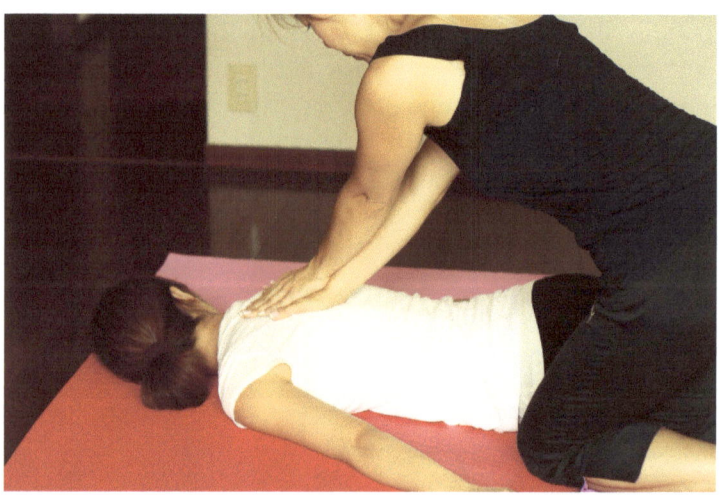

Melting Hardness in the Shoulder Blades

Hardness or tension in the shoulder blades affects the entire arm, blocking energy flow through the arm meridians, especially those of the lung and large intestine. There is also a point in the middle of the shoulder blade corresponding to the small intestine. It is known as "Ten So," or Small Intestine 11. It was used to relieve chest pain, as well as neck and shoulder stiffness and lack of strength in the arms. To activate energy in the shoulder blades, place both hands on either side as shown below. Use the thumbs, fingertips, and base of the palms to actively massage. Continue for about one minute, losening any tension in the surrounding muscles and tendons while sending energy from the center of the palms to the small intestine points on both sides.

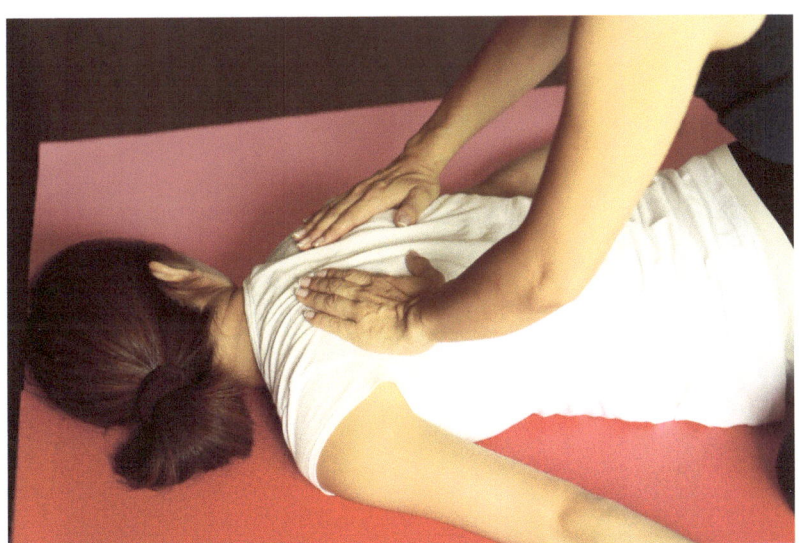

Energizing the Lower Back

The lower back is a frequent site of stress and tension. Many people hold tightness here. This region corresponds to the kidneys and intestines. Massaging the lower back soothes and stimulates these vital organs. The technique is simple. Place both hands across the spine as shown below. Place your thumbs on one side of the spine and your fingers on the other side. Use a deep kneading motion to massage this area. This proccedure loosens stagnation in the kidneys and adrenal glands and activates the smooth flow of energy in the intestines. Problems in the kidneys often result from too much animal protein, fat, salt, and chilled beverages.

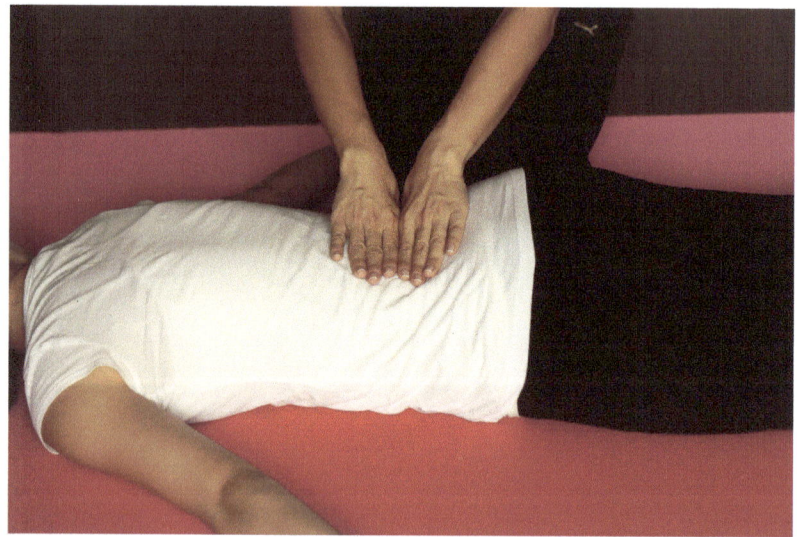

Clearing Stagnation in the Buttocks

To massage the buttocks, move slightly downward so that you can reach the indented area in the center of both sides of the buttock. Place the base of your palms firmly in this area and massage with an upward and outward circular motion. Repeat for about one minute. This is helpful in activating organs in the lower body, including the intestines, bladder, and reproductive organs, while strengthening overall vitality, especially in the legs.

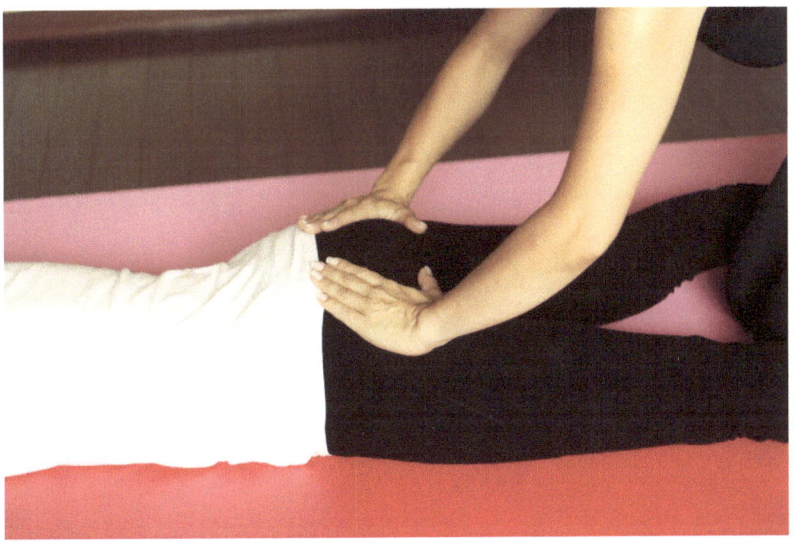

Equalizing Left and Right

In most cases, the legs are not perfectly even. If one is longer than the other, it indicates imbalance between the left and right sides of the body. This can affect the flow of energy in the body as a whole. It may also indicate that the pelvis is slanted in the direction of the longer leg; the result of overexpansion in the organs on that side, especially the kidneys, intestines, and sexual organs. To help correct this imbalance, grasp both ankles as shown below. Gently pull both legs slightly upward and outward, lower them back to the ground, and slowly release. Repeat several times. This helps rebalance the energy flowing through the lower body organs and meridians of the leg.

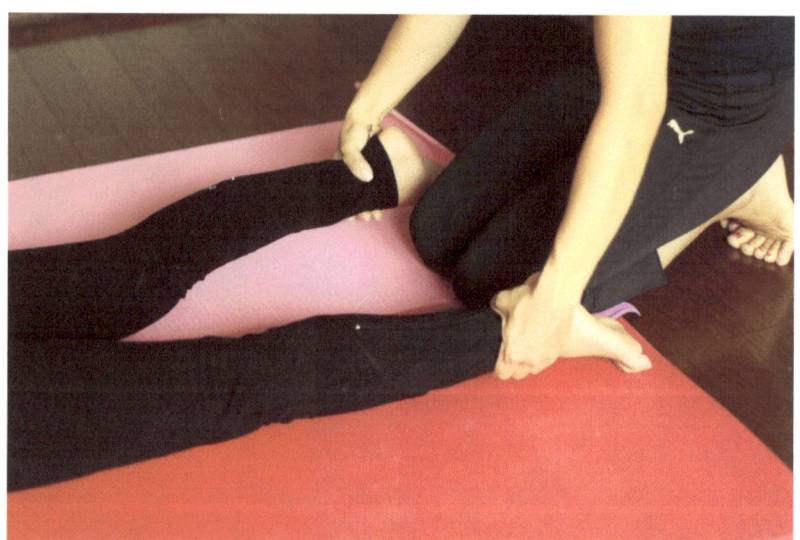

Stretching the Legs

To stretch and release stagnation in the leg meridians, and in the muscles and joints, grasp both ankles as shown below. Bend the legs at the knee, cross the feet at the ankles, and press down toward the buttocks. Return the legs to an upright position, reverse the feet and again press toward the buttocks. After you finish, return the feet to the floor. Note: don't force the feet toward the buttocks but stop pushing once resistance is encountered. Also, do not perform this exercise on those with stiff, painful, or inflamed joints.

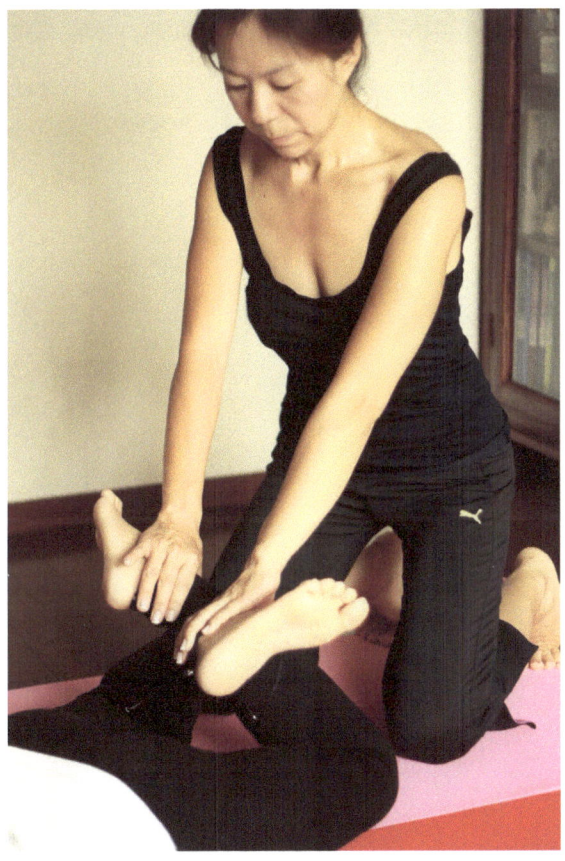

Massaging the Legs

The bladder meridian runs down the back of both legs in the center. It ends in the fifth toe. Together with the kidney meridian, which runs up the inside of the leg, the bladder meridian helps control the vertical flow of energy through the entire body. This meridian can be energized and harmonized by gently massaging down the back of both legs. We massage both legs at the same time. Place your palms in the center of the legs with your thumbs and fingers outstretched. Starting at the top, begin a gentle kneading motion. Gradually work your way from the top down to the ankle, maintaining an even rhythm with your thumbs, palms, and fingers. Repeat several times until stress and tension are eased.

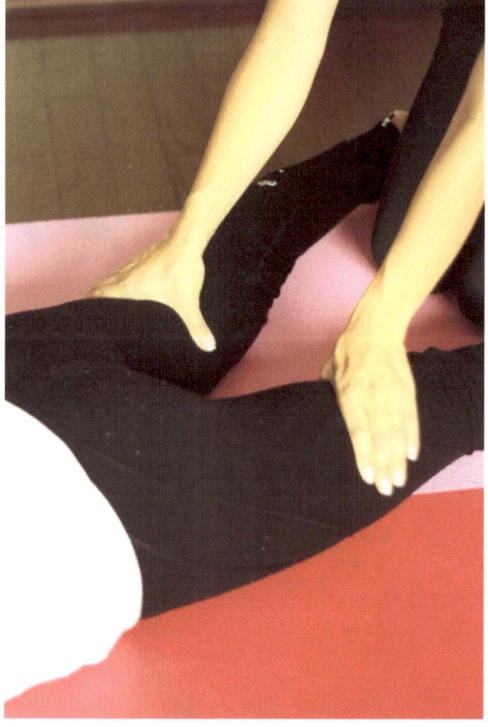

Foot Massage

As reflexologists know, the foot has correspondences with every part of the body. The feet and toes contain key points that energize the organs and meridians. Perhaps the most well known of these is Kidney 1 located in the ball of the foot.

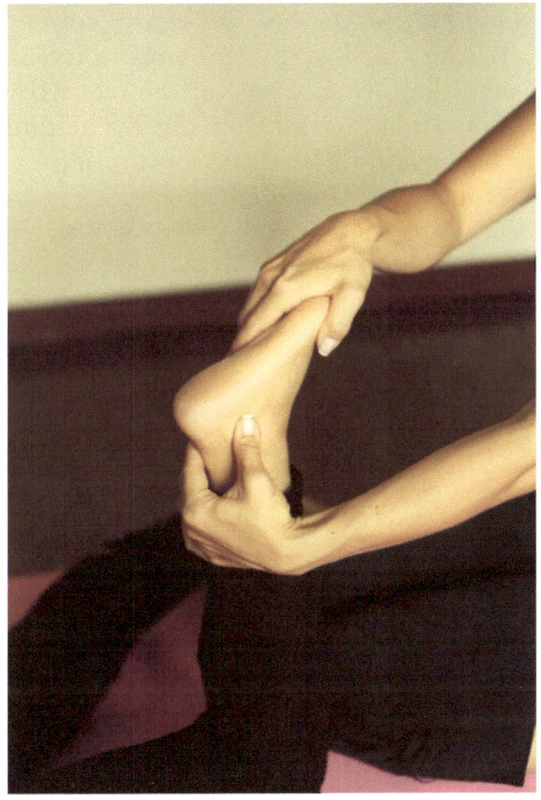

There are numerous techniques for massaging the foot that are helpful in activating and stimulating the body's energy. This exercise involves three steps. Begin by bending the leg at the knee so that the foot is raised for massage.

In the first step, grasp the toes and sole of the foot with your active hand, while grasping the ankle with your other hand for support. Begin to gently twirl and rotate the foot using the ankle as the axis of rotation. Go in one direction several times then reverse direction for several times. This loosens tension in the joint and relaxes the meridians that cross the ankle. In the second step, use your thumbs and fingers to massage the Achilles tendon using a gentle up and down motion. Repeat for a minute or two. This step activates the reproductive organs and kidneys. In the third step, use your active hand to rub and massage the toes and sole of the foot with a back and forth motion. Hold the foot steady by holding the ankle with your other hand. Continue for a minute or so or until the sole becomes warm and energized.

This activates the entire body as well as the meridians of the spleen, pancreas, and liver (first toe), stomach (second and third toes), gallbladder (fourth toe), bladder (fifth toe), and kidney (bottom of the foot.) Perform these steps on one side. Return the foot to the resting position on the floor. Then repeat on the other side, returning the foot to the resting position once the steps are completed.

Easing Tension in the Arms

The arm is the channel for six meridians. On the inside of the arm the lung, heart governor (body circulation), and heart meridians run from the body out to the fingers. On the outside of the arm, the large intestine, triple heater (body metabolism centered in the thyroid), and small intestine meridians run from the fingers back toward the body.

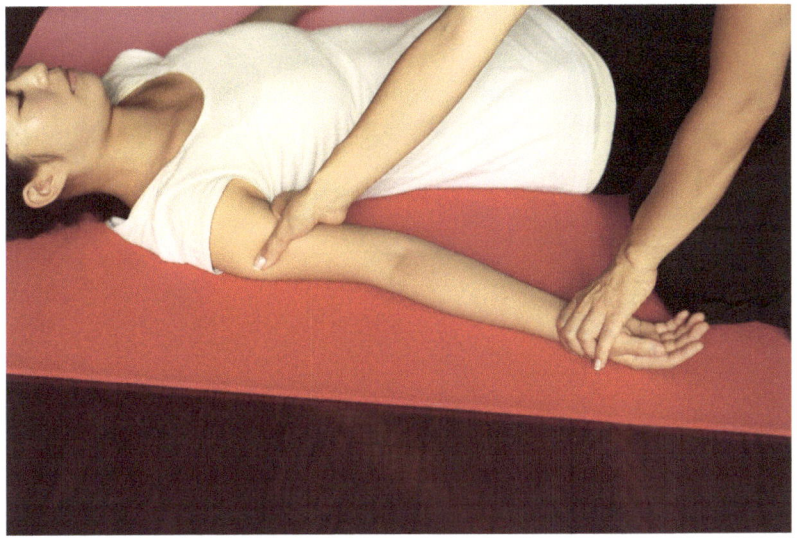

To perform this step, as well as the steps that follow, ask the receiver to turn over so that he or she is lying comfortably on the back with arms extended slightly to the sides. (Before proceeding to the arms, you have the option to massage the front of the legs, using the method described in the leg massage section. In this case, position your hands across the front of the legs above both ankles and massage upwards in sections, pausing after each section, and from the ankles to the pelvis. Both legs can be done at the same time.)

To massage the three inner meridians and also relax the muscles and tendons in the arm, place your active hand across the inside of the arm just below the armpit, with your thumb and fingers positioned opposite to each other. Grasp the wrist with your other hand for support. Using a gentle squeezing motion, press down the inside of the arm from the armpit to the wrist, one section at a time.

Squeeze, release, and move to the next section, repeating until you reach the wrist. Repeat several times. Then, flip the arm over and repeat the procedure on the outside, however, in this case, massage up the arm in the opposite direction, so as to follow meridian flow on the outside of the arm. Repeat several times. Before you do the other arm, first massage the hand as described in the next section.

Hand Massage

Like the foot, the hand, especially the palm and fingers, has correspondences with the entire body. As we saw in the previous step, three meridians run along the inner arm to the fingers. The meridian correspondences include the thumb – lungs, index finger – large intestine, middle finger – heart governor, ring finger – triple heater, and little finger – heart (inside) and small intestine (outside.)

To massage the hands, place the receiver's hand on your knee. Place your fingers under the hand for support while keeping both thumbs free for massage. Begin to massage the palm by pressing your thumbs rapidly, one after the other, into the palm, working your way around the entire palm. During the massage, press the area in the center of the palm. This point is known as Heart Governor 8. Massaging it activates circulation and overall vitality.

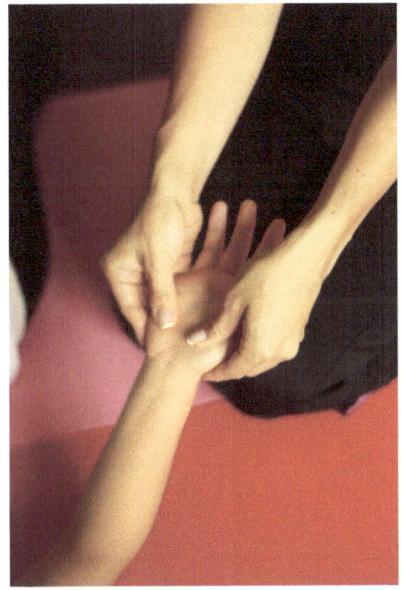

Extend your massage to each of the fingers beginning with the thumb. Repeatedly press each finger, starting at the base and working outward. Repeat several times. Before finishing you have the option to turn the hand over, exposing the other side. Use your thumb to massage the area between the thumb and index finger. This point is known as Large Intestine 4 and is important for many reasons, including activating and energizing the large intestine.

Once these steps are completed, return the receiver's hand to the floor. Move to the opposite side of the receiver and repeat, beginning with the arm, as outlined in the previous section, and finishing with the hand and fingers.

Massaging the Colon

Pain or hardness in the large intestine is often a sign of constipation and irregularity. Gentle massage offers a simple method to bring relief. Sit alongside the receiver so that you can comfortably reach the abdomen. Place the fingers of your active hand together and extend them outward. Extend the fingers of your other hand and place it on top for support. Place the tips of your extended fingers on the lower right abdomen (the beginning of the ascending colon.) Breathe together with the receiver several times, and on the final exhale, press gently into the abdomen. Then inhale together and slowly release pressure. Reposition your hands further up the right side and repeat. Repeat along the entire length of the colon, continuing up the right, across the center beneath the ribcage, and down the left side to the pelvis. The entire procedure can be repeated several times.

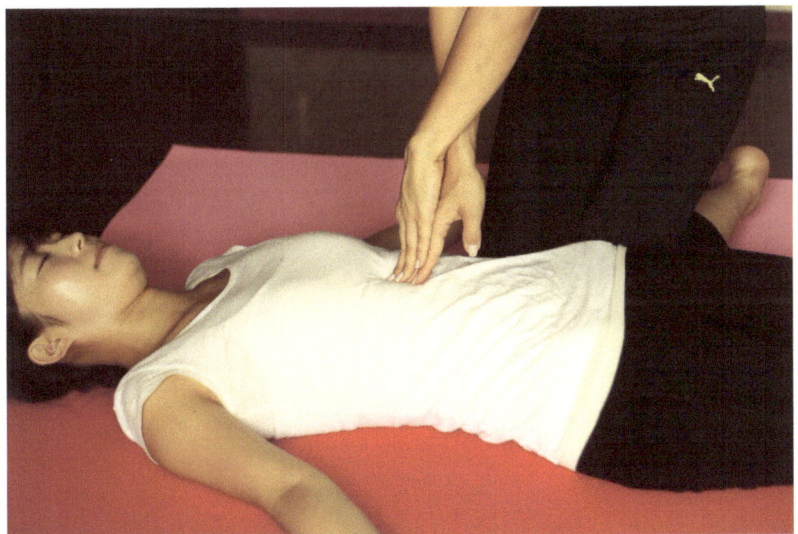

Hara Massage

In Japan, the region deep within the small intestine is referred to as "hara." Located about three fingers below the navel, it is considered the vital center of the body. In Chinese it is referred to as the "lower dantian," and in yoga philosophy as the "swadhisthana chakra," the seat of prana (energy) that radiates outward to the whole body. Hara is the site where nutrients are absorbed into the bloodstream. Simple massage on the hara helps strengthen this function and improve vitality in general. Place both hands across the abdomen with fingers extended. Begin to massage with a gentle kneading motion, rocking slightly back and forth. Continue for about a minute or two until the region becomes relaxed and energized.

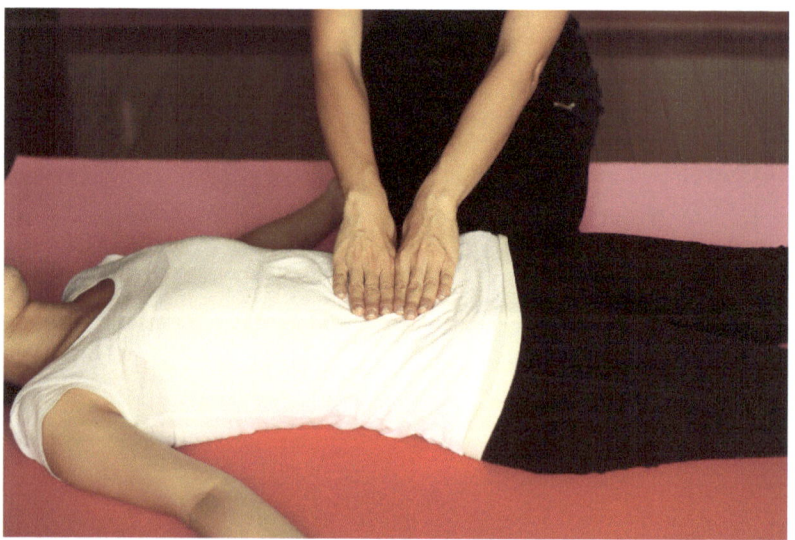

Relaxing the Face

The facial muscles are often tense due to poor diet and the stress of modern life. To help release this tension, sit above the receiver's head and place both palms on the cheeks with your fingers extended. Hold your hands in this position for about a minute, and coordinate your breathing with that of the receiver. Breathe in a relaxed and gentle rhythm. Once your energies are harmonized, gently rub the cheeks up and down until they become warm. (You can also massage the ears. Grasp both ears with the thumbs and index fingers. Gently massage beginning at the top and working your way down to the lobes. Repeat several times. Then place your hands back on the cheeks.) Return to the still position and breathe together for a minute or two before slowly removing your hands.

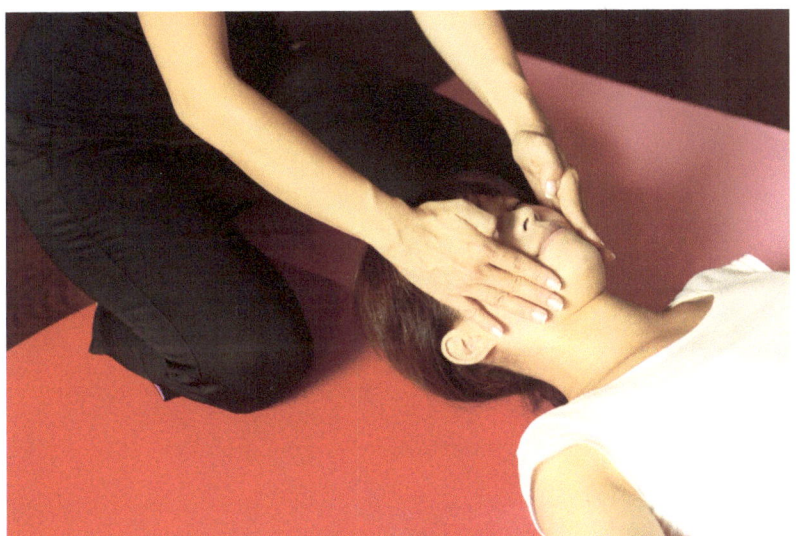

ABOUT THE AUTHORS

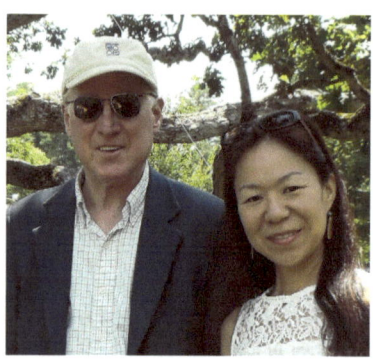

Edward Esko is one of the world's leading teachers and counselors on the macrobiotic way of life. He studied with Michio Kushi for many years and has served as Executive Director of the East West Foundation in Boston and Director of the Kushi Institute of the Berkshires. Edward is a co-founder and Board member of Planetary Health, Inc. He has personally counseled and guided thousands of people toward improved health and well-being. Edward founded the International Macrobiotic Institute in 2016 to further the dream and vision of his mentor, Michio Kushi, and to make quality macrobiotic education and guidance available to people around the world. He is author of *Basic Shiatsu, Ki: The Energy of Life,* and many other titles.

Naomi Ichikawa Esko is a 2010 graduate of the Kushi Institute (K.I.) in Massachusetts. Prior to her study at the K.I. she worked in the restaurant industry in her native Tokyo. In 2011 she established an educational center known as Macrobiotics Japan. Naomi also managed a consulting business advising restaurants in the preparation of healthy menus. She lives in Western Mass. with her husband. Naomi is the author of *Smart Vegan: Recipes from Naomi's Kitchen* published in 2017 by IMI Press.

Contact: International Macrobiotic Institute (IMI)
P.O. Box 2051
Lenox, Massachusetts 01240
InternationalMacrobioticInstitute.com

---

www.ingramcontent.com/pod-product-compliance
Lightning Source LLC
Chambersburg PA
CBHW050921290526
45792CB00002B/848